Post-Incid Recovery Considerations of the Health Care Service Delivery Infrastructure

Workshop Summary

Theresa Wizemann and Bruce M. Altevogt,
Rapporteurs

Forum on Medical and Public Health Preparedness for
Catastrophic Events

Board on Health Sciences Policy

INSTITUTE OF MEDICINE
OF THE NATIONAL ACADEMIES

THE NATIONAL ACADEMIES PRESS
Washington, D.C.
www.nap.edu

THE NATIONAL ACADEMIES PRESS • 500 Fifth Street, NW • Washington, DC 20001

NOTICE: The project that is the subject of this report was approved by the Governing Board of the National Research Council, whose members are drawn from the councils of the National Academy of Sciences, the National Academy of Engineering, and the Institute of Medicine. The members of the committee responsible for the report were chosen for their special competences and with regard for appropriate balance.

This study was supported by contracts between the National Academy of Sciences and the American College of Emergency Physicians; American Hospital Association; American Medical Association; American Nurses Association; Association of State and Territorial Health Officials; Centers for Disease Control and Prevention (Contract No. 200-2005-13434 TO #6); Department of the Army (Contract No. W81XWH-08-P-0934); Department of Health and Human Services' National Institutes of Health (Contract No. N01-OD-4-2139 TO #198 and TO #244); Department of Health and Human Services' Office of the Assistant Secretary for Preparedness and Response (Contract Nos. HHSP233200900680P, HHS P23320042509X1); Department of Homeland Security's Federal Emergency Management Agency (Contract No. HSFEHQ-08-P-1800); Department of Homeland Security's Office of Health Affairs (Contract No. HSHQDC-07-C-00097); Department of Transportation's National Highway Traffic Safety Administration (Contract No. DTNH22-10-H-00287); Department of Veterans Affairs (Contract No. V101(93)P-2136 TO #10); Emergency Nurses Association; National Association of Chain Drug Stores; National Association of County and City Health Officials; National Association of Emergency Medical Technicians; Pharmaceutical Research and Manufacturers of America; Robert Wood Johnson Foundation; and United Health Foundation. The views presented in this publication do not necessarily reflect the views of the organizations or agencies that provided support for the project.

International Standard Book Number-13: 978-0-309-26060-2
International Standard Book Number-10: 0-309-26060-4

Additional copies of this report are available for sale from the National Academies Press, 500 Fifth Street, NW, Keck 360, Washington, DC 20001; (800) 624-6242 or (202) 334-3313; http://www.nap.edu/.

For more information about the Institute of Medicine, visit the IOM home page at: **www.iom.edu.**

The serpent has been a symbol of long life, healing, and knowledge among almost all cultures and religions since the beginning of recorded history. The serpent adopted as a logotype by the Institute of Medicine is a relief carving from ancient Greece, now held by the Staatliche Museen in Berlin.

Suggested citation: IOM (Institute of Medicine). 2012. *Post-incident recovery considerations of the health care service delivery infrastructure: Workshop summary.* Washington, DC: The National Academies Press.

"Knowing is not enough; we must apply.
Willing is not enough; we must do."
—Goethe

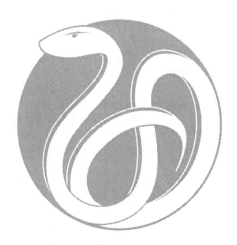

INSTITUTE OF MEDICINE
OF THE NATIONAL ACADEMIES

Advising the Nation. Improving Health.

THE NATIONAL ACADEMIES
Advisers to the Nation on Science, Engineering, and Medicine

The **National Academy of Sciences** is a private, nonprofit, self-perpetuating society of distinguished scholars engaged in scientific and engineering research, dedicated to the furtherance of science and technology and to their use for the general welfare. Upon the authority of the charter granted to it by the Congress in 1863, the Academy has a mandate that requires it to advise the federal government on scientific and technical matters. Dr. Ralph J. Cicerone is president of the National Academy of Sciences.

The **National Academy of Engineering** was established in 1964, under the charter of the National Academy of Sciences, as a parallel organization of outstanding engineers. It is autonomous in its administration and in the selection of its members, sharing with the National Academy of Sciences the responsibility for advising the federal government. The National Academy of Engineering also sponsors engineering programs aimed at meeting national needs, encourages education and research, and recognizes the superior achievements of engineers. Dr. Charles M. Vest is president of the National Academy of Engineering.

The **Institute of Medicine** was established in 1970 by the National Academy of Sciences to secure the services of eminent members of appropriate professions in the examination of policy matters pertaining to the health of the public. The Institute acts under the responsibility given to the National Academy of Sciences by its congressional charter to be an adviser to the federal government and, upon its own initiative, to identify issues of medical care, research, and education. Dr. Harvey V. Fineberg is president of the Institute of Medicine.

The **National Research Council** was organized by the National Academy of Sciences in 1916 to associate the broad community of science and technology with the Academy's purposes of furthering knowledge and advising the federal government. Functioning in accordance with general policies determined by the Academy, the Council has become the principal operating agency of both the National Academy of Sciences and the National Academy of Engineering in providing services to the government, the public, and the scientific and engineering communities. The Council is administered jointly by both Academies and the Institute of Medicine. Dr. Ralph J. Cicerone and Dr. Charles M. Vest are chair and vice chair, respectively, of the National Research Council.

PLANNING COMMITTEE ON LONG-TERM RECOVERY OF THE HEALTH CARE SERVICE DELIVERY INFRASTRUCTURE[1]

JACK HERRMANN (*Co-Chair*), National Association of County and City Health Officials, Washington, DC
LYNNE KIDDER (*Co-Chair*), Bipartisan WMD Terrorism Research Center, Washington, DC

Project Staff

BRUCE M. ALTEVOGT, Preparedness Forum Director
KRISTIN VISWANATHAN, Research Associate (until June 2012)
ALEX REPACE, Senior Program Assistant
ANDREW M. POPE, Director, Board on Health Sciences Policy

---

[1]Institute of Medicine planning committees are solely responsible for organizing the workshop, identifying topics, and choosing speakers. The responsibility for the published workshop summary rests with the workshop rapporteurs and the institution.

v

FORUM ON MEDICAL AND PUBLIC HEALTH PREPAREDNESS FOR CATASTROPHIC EVENTS[1]

ROBERT KADLEC (*Co-Chair*), PRTM Management Consultants, Washington, DC

LYNNE KIDDER (*Co-Chair*), Bipartisan WMD Terrorism Research Center, Washington, DC

ALEX ADAMS, National Association of Chain Drug Stores Foundation, Alexandria, VA

GEORGES BENJAMIN, American Public Health Association, Washington, DC

D. W. CHEN, Office of Assistant Secretary of Defense for Health Affairs, Department of Defense, Washington, DC (since June 2012)

BROOKE COURTNEY, Food and Drug Administration, Silver Spring, MD

JEFFREY DUCHIN, Seattle & King County and University of Washington

ALEXANDER GARZA, Department of Homeland Security, Washington, DC

JULIE GERBERDING, Merck Vaccines, West Point, PA

LEWIS GOLDFRANK, New York University Medical Center, NY

DAN HANFLING, Inova Health System, Falls Church, VA

JACK HERRMANN, National Association of County and City Health Officials, Washington, DC

JAMES JAMES, American Medical Association, Chicago, IL

PAUL JARRIS, Association of State and Territorial Health Officials, Arlington, VA

JERRY JOHNSTON, National Association of Emergency Medical Technicians, Mt. Pleasant, IA (until January 2012)

BRIAN KAMOIE, The White House, Washington, DC

LISA KAPLOWITZ, Department of Health and Human Sciences Office of the Assistant Secretary for Preparedness and Response, Washington, DC

ALI KHAN, Centers for Disease Control and Prevention, Atlanta, GA

MICHAEL KURILLA, National Institute of Allergy and Infectious Diseases, Bethesda, MD

JAYNE LUX, National Business Group on Health, Washington, DC

---

[1]Institute of Medicine forums and roundtables do not issue, review, or approve individual documents. The responsibility for the published workshop summary rests with the workshop rapporteurs and the institution.

ANTHONY MacINTYRE, American College of Emergency Physicians, Washington, DC

NICOLE McKOIN, Target Corporation, Minneapolis, MN (from April 2012)

MARGARET McMAHON, Emergency Nurses Association, Williamstown, NJ

MATTHEW MINSON, Texas A&M University, College Station

ERIN MULLEN, Pharmaceutical Research and Manufacturers of America, Washington, DC

CHERYL PETERSON, American Nurses Association, Silver Spring, MD

STEVEN PHILLIPS, National Library of Medicine, Bethesda, MD

LEWIS RADONOVICH, Veterans Health Administration, Washington, DC

JOSHUA RIFF, Target Corporation, Minneapolis, MN (until April 2012)

KENNETH SCHOR, Uniformed Services University of the Health Sciences, Bethesda, MD (from April 2012)

ROSLYNE SCHULMAN, American Hospital Association, Washington, DC

SARAH SEILER, Carolinas Medical Center, Charlotte, NC

RICHARD SERINO, Federal Emergency Management Agency, Washington, DC

MICHAEL SKIDMORE, U.S. Department of Defense, Washington, DC (until May 2012)

SHARON STANLEY, American Red Cross, Washington, DC

ERIC TONER, University of Pittsburgh Medical Center, PA

REED TUCKSON, UnitedHealth Group, Minneapolis, MN

MARGARET VANAMRINGE, The Joint Commission, Washington, DC

GAMUNU WIEJETUNGE, National Highway Traffic Safety Administration, Washington, DC

IOM Staff

BRUCE ALTEVOGT, Project Director

KRISTIN VISWANATHAN, Research Associate (until June 2012)

ALEX REPACE, Senior Program Assistant

ANDREW M. POPE, Director, Board on Health Sciences Policy

Reviewers

This workshop summary has been reviewed in draft form by individuals chosen for their diverse perspectives and technical expertise, in accordance with procedures approved by the National Research Council's Report Review Committee. The purpose of this independent review is to provide candid and critical comments that will assist the institution in making its published summary as sound as possible and to ensure that the summary meets institutional standards for objectivity, evidence, and responsiveness to the study charge. The review comments and draft manuscript remain confidential to protect the integrity of the process. We wish to thank the following individuals for their review of this summary:

James Craig, Mississippi State Department of Health
Onora Lien, King County Healthcare Coalition
Rev. Kevin Massey, Advocate Lutheran General Hospital
Linda Williams, Montana State University, Chouteau County
  Extension

Although the reviewers listed above have provided many constructive comments and suggestions, they did not see the final draft of the workshop summary before its release. The review of this summary was overseen by **Kristine M. Gebbie,** Flinders University School of Nursing and Midwifery. Appointed by the Institute of Medicine, she was responsible for making certain that an independent examination of this workshop summary was carried out in accordance with institutional procedures and that all review comments were carefully considered. Responsibility for the final content of this summary rests entirely with the workshop rapporteurs and the institution.

Contents

REFERENCE

APPENDIXES

Workshop Summary

INTRODUCTION

As part of its ongoing mission to foster dialogue among stakeholders and to confront the challenges inherent in ensuring the nation's health security, the Institute of Medicine (IOM) Forum on Medical and Public Health Preparedness for Catastrophic Events sponsored a town hall session at the 2012 Public Health Preparedness Summit, held February 21-24 in Anaheim, California.[1] The session was facilitated by Lynne Kidder, president of the Bipartisan WMD Terrorism Research Center and co-chair of the IOM Forum.

As summarized by Kidder, other sessions of the 2012 Summit discussed the value of regional capacity building; the importance of interagency, intergovernmental, and public-private collaboration; and the significant role that health care coalitions can play in ensuring resilient communities and national health security. In this session sponsored by the IOM, the focus of discussion was sustaining health care delivery beyond the initial response to a disaster and facilitating the full long-term recovery of the local health care delivery systems. The following text serves as a summary of only the IOM-sponsored session.

As part of the critical infrastructure of any community, health systems and assets are vital not only for the safety and well-being of its citizens, but also for the economic vitality, quality of life, and livelihood

---

[1]The planning committee's role was limited to planning the town hall session, i.e., workshop. The summary has been prepared by the workshop rapporteurs as a factual summary of what occurred at the workshop. Statements, recommendations, and opinions expressed are those of individual presenters and participants, and are not necessarily endorsed or verified by the IOM, and they should not be construed as reflecting any group consensus.

of the entire community. Many elements required for recovery are also fundamental to the day-to-day operations of these systems (e.g., information sharing, identifying and leveraging existing capabilities of medical providers in a community, developing trusted relationships). Investing in improved health care delivery systems, both financially and through collaborative capacity building, can enhance economic development and growth before a disaster, and also prove instrumental in sustaining services and recovering after a disaster.

While the impacted local communities are the first responders and the drivers of long-term recovery, this session also discussed the important supportive roles played by the federal government, the private sector, nongovernmental organizations (NGOs), and state officials. Specifically, the session was designed to engage representatives from federal, state, and local governments, and the nonprofit and private sectors to do the following:

- Identify services necessary to maintain or improve the affected health care service delivery infrastructure to ensure it meets the long-term physical and behavioral health needs of affected populations.
- Discuss the roles and functions of the relevant Recovery Support Functions in facilitating long-term recovery of the health care service delivery infrastructure.
- Highlight lessons learned from previous disasters, and identify priorities for pre-incident operational plans, with a specific focus on opportunities to leverage programs and activities across the public, private, and nonprofit sectors that support long-term recovery and mass casualty care.

This report summarizes the presentations and commentary by the invited panelists.[2]

---

[2]The complete statement of task can be found in Appendix A.

THE FEDERAL GOVERNMENT: COORDINATOR AND FACILITATOR

The National Disaster Recovery Framework

The National Disaster Recovery Framework (NDRF) was released in September 2011 by the Federal Emergency Management Administration (FEMA), in collaboration with other federal partners, following a series of information-gathering public meetings across the country. Deborah Ingram, assistant administrator for the Recovery Directorate of FEMA, explained that the NDRF is one of a series of integrated national planning frameworks covering prevention, protection, mitigation, response, and recovery that are required under Presidential Policy Directive-8 on national preparedness.

The NDRF establishes a powerful mechanism to support recovery problem solving, improve access to resources, and foster coordination among state, tribal, territorial, and federal agencies and nongovernmental organization (NGO) partners and stakeholders. This represents a new way of thinking about managing disasters, Ingram said. Although much focus has been on response, those initial activities that are critical to saving lives and property, even more work needs to be done beyond that. The NDRF provides common language and concepts to foster full community-based recovery. "Whole community," Ingram explained, includes all levels of government, the private sector, nonprofit and faith-based organizations, and others in the community, working together to help support the recovery process. The NDRF is a national framework in the sense that it is national in scope and community-based; it is not a federal framework (i.e., for how the federal government will manage recovery). Decisions need to be made at the community level about how best to move forward for each community. As FEMA looks at recovery, it is going beyond FEMA, Ingram said. The framework is not about new authorities and new funding—it is about leveraging existing resources and understanding how to deploy them more effectively.

The NDRF defines roles and responsibilities and promotes establishment of post-disaster organizations to support recovery. It is scalable and flexible, and provides for a deliberate and transparent process.

The three key elements of the NDRF are

- **Planning**—both pre- and post-disaster recovery planning.
- **Leadership**—at the local, state, tribal, and federal levels.

- **Recovery Support Functions**—working with federal partners to provide structure for communities, states, and tribes to use in pre- and post-disaster planning and recovery efforts. The six functional areas of assistance are described in Box 1.

BOX 1
Recovery Support Functions (Lead Coordinating Agency)

Community Planning and Capacity Building (FEMA)
- Helping the community bring its stakeholders together to establish the vision, priorities, goals, and milestones for that community.

Economic (U.S. Department of Commerce)
- Fostering the ability to sustain the community through the workforce (e.g., having a tax base in the community that supports community services, having places for people to buy food so that they will stay in the community).

Health and Social Services (U.S. Department of Health and Human Services)
- Focused on the restoration of health and social services.

Housing (U.S. Department of Housing and Urban Development)
- Supporting a state-led housing task force to address housing needs, particularly rebuilding post-disaster.

Infrastructure (U.S. Army Corps of Engineers)
- Recovery of systems such as roads, bridges, power, and transportation. Minimizing disruption, ensuring access to health facilities and other necessary functions.

Natural and Cultural Resources (U.S. Department of Interior)
- Minimizing the harm to and facilitating the recovery of resources that are vital to the identity of communities (e.g., wetlands, parks, historic monuments, properties).

SOURCE: Ingram presentation (February 23, 2012).

Playing a key role to support the NDRF are the Federal Disaster Recovery Coordinators. Coordinators are responsible for working with the state, tribe, or local community to identify its recovery needs and convene the necessary recovery support functions. Ingram noted that

FEMA is currently hiring for these positions and is planning to have one coordinator in each of the 10 FEMA regional offices to support pre-disaster planning in the states.

Using the Health and Social Services Recovery Support Function as an example, Ingram illustrated how the functions work together to promote optimally coordinated assistance. Other functions that may be critical to the success of the Health and Social Services function are the Infrastructure function, which helps to provide timely and well-prioritized access to hospitals; the Economic function, which may be instrumental in the rebuilding of private health care facilities; the Community Planning and Capacity Building function, which brings the whole-community view to comprehensive recovery planning and supports the identification of priorities; and the Housing function, which informs where residential areas might be established, or where health care needs can be anticipated.

Effective coordination is essential for effective disaster assistance, for the health care sector as well as all sectors, Ingram concluded. The NDRF provides the necessary planning, coordination, leadership, and structure to allow that to happen. It is early in the process, Ingram noted, but as the NDRF moves ahead, we will start to see communities thinking more about the recovery process, bringing in partners, building networks in advance, and working together in a pre-disaster setting to plan how best to manage post-disaster needs.

Office of the Assistant Secretary for Preparedness and Response—Portal to the Full Spectrum of Department of Health and Human Services (HHS) Resources

In addition to the partnership with FEMA on the NDRF described by Ingram, HHS collaborates with the Department of Defense, the Department of Homeland Security, the Department of Veterans Affairs, the Department of Commerce, and a host of other interagency partners on recovery activities, said Kevin Yeskey, Deputy Assistant Secretary for Preparedness and Response and director of the Office of Preparedness and Emergency Operations in the HHS Office of the Assistant Secretary for Preparedness and Response (ASPR).

As one example of a response and recovery planning program at ASPR, Yeskey described the Hospital Preparedness Program (HPP). One aspect of the program is the development of health care service resilience through hospital coalitions. If a hospital becomes incapacitated or destroyed (e.g., as happened in Joplin, Missouri, in May 2011 as the result of an EF-5 tornado) there will be other hospitals in that community that are prepared to assist with pre-established Memorandums of Understanding (MOUs) and agreements that facilitate the sharing of resources and care of patients. The HPP also supports hospital and medical facilities in the development of continuity-of-operations plans. It is much easier for facilities to shelter-in-place if they can than to evacuate and move patients, Yeskey said. Administratively, it is easier to keep operational at some level than it is to shut down and reopen at a later time. Another focus of HPP is medical surge capabilities, for example, the availability of mobile facilities.

With regard to disaster response, the resources of the entire HHS department are engaged and committed, including, for example, the Centers for Disease Control and Prevention (CDC), Food and Drug Administration, National Institutes of Health (NIH), Health Resources and Services Administration, Substance Abuse and Mental Health Services Administration, Centers for Medicare & Medicaid Services (CMS), Administration for Children and Families, and ASPR. It is not just ASPR and the National Disaster Medical System involved in response, Yeskey stressed, but the entire HHS department. When it comes to recovery, HHS also wants to have the entire department applying its existing authorities, regulations, and resources to assist in the recovery effort, he said. For both response and recovery, ASPR provides "one-stop shopping" for communities in need to muster the resources of the entire HHS department.

Some of the most common questions, and also some of the most complex, that ASPR receives concern hospital and health care facility reimbursement under disaster conditions. Can we bill for care that was provided in a tent? Or bill for services provided in a modular facility we built that is licensed by the state? Answers to these complex and nuanced questions vary somewhat from situation to situation, and addressing them is a part of continuity-of-operations planning. In the past 4 or 5 years, Yeskey noted, CMS has become very engaged in response and recovery and has been proactive in trying to address these needs through its regional offices. For example, CMS has posted answers to "frequently asked questions" about reimbursement issues on its website, and makes staff available to assist with issues and waivers.

Another important resource is the authority of the Secretary of HHS to declare a public health emergency, commented Yeskey. This allows the Secretary to take certain actions and waive certain requirements or sanctions. When the President has also declared an emergency or disaster, the Secretary may apply certain waivers under section 1135 of the Social Security Act. For example, the Secretary can waive certain sanctions or penalties for not adhering to certain provisions of laws, such as the Health Insurance Portability and Accountability Act (HIPAA) or the Emergency Medical Treatment and Labor Act (EMTALA), during the declared emergency and for a specified period of time. This gives facilities some flexibility and reduces their administrative burden, so that patients can be taken care of in a timely fashion.

Yeskey reiterated Ingram's comments that as the lead agency for the Health and Social Services Recovery Support Function, the whole of HHS is engaged to support locally led recovery efforts and restoration of public health, health care, and social services. This also includes behavioral health, environmental health, food safety, school impacts, and long-term health of responders.

HHS is working to make response and recovery a seamless transition, and Yeskey encouraged participants to get to know their own regional emergency coordinators, who work in every HHS region throughout the country.

THE PRIVATE SECTOR: BUILDING RESILIENT COMMUNITIES

The private sector has an important role to play in preparing for and responding to public health emergencies and in building resilient communities. Joshua Riff, chief medical officer at Target Corporation, explained how Target is actively involved in building public–private relationships to improve community preparedness and public health response.

Sharing Our Strengths

Target is a Fortune 30 company employing 360,000 team members. More than 25 million guests visit every week, generating $62 billion in annual sales. Headquartered in Minnesota with international offices in over 20 countries, Target is the fifth-largest U.S. retailer, with more than 1,740 stores and 38 distribution centers in 49 states. Riff stressed that Target is more than simply a merchandiser (i.e., involved in sales and promotion of products). Target Corporation is also a retailer (i.e., buys goods in large quantities and maintains a robust supply chain), as well as food supplier, pharmacy, bank, credit card issuer, health care provider, and employer. The company needs to protect all of these businesses in the same way that others in the community need to protect their businesses. By partnering together, Riff said, we can share our stories and our strengths.

Target is committed to the health and well-being of communities, both every day and in response to public health emergencies, and is an active partner with many health-related agencies throughout the country. Disaster preparedness, relief, and recovery are top priorities for the company as they work to protect Target team members, guests, and businesses, as well as contributing to the resiliencies of communities. Riff added that Target looks at these public partnerships as a public good, not as a competitive advantage. The company is able to respond when asked for drug distribution or immunizations because it has such a large U.S. presence, but Walgreens, CVS, Wal-Mart, or other competitors complement Target's footprint, he said, and Target will bring them to the table as well.

As an example of Target's commitment to public well-being, Riff described the company's comprehensive global crisis management program, which, he noted, is somewhat unique to Target. A key focus of the program is preparedness, including practice drills for emergency scenarios. A 24/7 Corporate Command Center at the headquarters in Minnesota, the "C3," tracks natural disasters around the world and alerts team members, partners, and vendors to developing situations and potential needs. There is also a global security program, and Target has extensive public safety partnerships with law enforcement, emergency management, and the public health sector as well as structures in place to respond to any major crisis affecting the company's businesses throughout the world. These partnerships are essential for Target's planning and preparedness, Riff said.

The Power of Planning Together

Riff emphasized that a response is much more robust when we prepare, plan, and exercise with our partners. For example, every year before hurricane season Target prepares its distribution centers by moving goods or services generally needed in hurricanes for easy mobilization. When a natural disaster is emerging as a threat to an area, the company ships all the supplies the local Target will need to protect its guests and team members and their communities, and to supply the public health partners in the area.

In 2011 during Hurricane Irene, 222 Target stores and distribution centers and many team members were in the path of the storm. In preparation for the storm, 117 stores closed. Of those, 109 stores and 3 distribution centers were impacted. Through multiple preparation calls, the Corporate Command Center advised stores on how to prepare their buildings, how to partner with local agencies, and most importantly, how to protect their team members and allow their team members to protect their homes and those of their friends and family (i.e., the community). The Corporate Command Center also helped to ensure that local management teams could get the support they needed.

Throughout a crisis, the Corporate Command Center keeps Target teams informed and safe, donates funds, and participates in the recovery efforts. After Hurricane Irene, Target donated over a quarter of a million dollars to the Red Cross, Salvation Army, and other local organizations, as well as in-kind donations of relief kits to victims and rescuers. The company also sent team members to volunteer in the impacted communities. Team members, Riff said, are actually some of the company's greatest assets in recovery and relief, volunteering out of the kindness of their hearts and lending tremendous support.

Pre-established relationships and joint planning are the key to successful public-private relationships, Riff said. For example, in 2009, Target signed an MOU to formalize the relationship between Target and the California Emergency Management Agency so that the company can be fully integrated into California's state planning efforts. This provides the state with direct access to Target's thought leaders and decision makers, who can assist with resources or logistical support. It also allows the company to be better prepared to deliver needed supplies such as water and relief kits. In addition to California, Target has MOUs with Maryland and New Jersey. The MOU establishes that Target will be part of the planning process and that there will be two-way information sharing before, during, and after a crisis.

NONGOVERNMENTAL ORGANIZATIONS: PROVIDING SUPPORT AND RELIEF

The American Red Cross

The American Red Cross is a volunteer-led humanitarian organization that provides relief to victims of disaster and helps people prevent, prepare, and respond to emergencies. The relationship of the American Red Cross and the federal government is unique, said Linda MacIntyre, chair of the Red Cross National Nursing Committee and assistant clinical professor at the University of California, San Francisco. The Red Cross is both an independent, nonprofit, charitable organization and a congressionally chartered organization. Under the charter, the Red Cross is expected to carry out certain responsibilities, including, for example, supporting the provisions of the Geneva Convention, providing family communications and other supports to the U.S. military, and maintaining a system of domestic and international disaster relief under the National Response Plan, which is coordinated by FEMA. Despite this close relationship with the federal government, the Red Cross is not a governmental agency and does not receive federal funding on a regular basis to carry out its services and programs.

Health is crucial in community resilience and response in a disaster, MacIntyre said. The Red Cross is in the community before, during, and after a disaster. Public health and emergency services that the Red Cross provides include, for example, general population shelters (serving individuals with chronic illness, functional and access needs, and many others), emergency aid stations, supportive counseling, assistance in reunification with families and friends, and outreach and condolence visits. The Red Cross also works to link families and caregivers with resources. Long after the emergency shelter is gone, the Red Cross is there to provide long-term individual and family services. This may include client case management, assistance with unmet needs, and health and human services provided directly and through other agencies and partnerships.

For disaster health services, Red Cross has an MOU with CDC to provide morbidity and mortality data. While this is a somewhat unusual obligation, MacIntyre noted, this health information is essential in terms of planning and responding. Other services include assisting the community in providing health care education, implementing preventative measures such as vaccination, and supporting public health departments with surveillance. Mental health recovery and resilience information tools and resources can be provided to school personnel, community members, mental health providers, community service providers, and other key stakeholders. In addition, psychological first aid and other resilience training can be provided to community members, and post-deployment support and training can be provided to disaster responders. Red Cross Biomedical Services provides blood and blood products as needed, working with the American Association of Blood Banks.

As a partner in response and recovery, the Red Cross offers scalability of operational response, from a single-family fire to flood damage or a series of hurricanes or tornadoes. Scalability is key, and operations move from local to regional to nationwide deployment as needed, and then back again to the chapter level for recovery. Because the Red Cross is part of the community, MacIntyre said, it is also part of the recovery.

Reaffirming the comments by the other panelists, MacIntyre said that whole-community planning and preparedness as well as partnerships are the critical components of success in long-term recovery of health services. In fulfilling its mission the Red Cross works closely with other NGOs, partnering with countless local and national organizations. MacIntyre shared one example of planning and partnership success. Shortly after 9/11, a severe ice storm hit the Kansas City area. The Red Cross had difficulty gathering volunteers to support the response because most of them were in New York City dealing with the aftermath of the terrorist attacks. Despite this and other challenges, agencies worked together afterward to problem-solve and coordinate services. As a result, after Hurricane Katrina, approximately 3,000 evacuees were served at a "one-stop shop" that included public health, faith-based organizations, nonprofit organizations, hospital personnel, pharmacists, and nurses. Nurses, for example, helped to coordinate complex health care needs such as ensuring people were able to receive their chemotherapy or dialysis.

In closing, MacIntyre shared that one of her goals as chair of the National Nursing Committee is to better represent the communities that the Red Cross serves through increased diversity, both internally with volunteer and paid staff and externally with partnerships. Research has shown, she said, that when we better represent the communities that we serve, better health outcomes result.

LOCAL AND STATE ROLES: THE COMMUNITY
AS THE LEAD

The new National Disaster Recovery Framework is helpful because it articulates things that have been needed at the state and local levels for quite some time, said James Craig, director of the Office of Health Protection at the Mississippi State Department of Health. The most effective, efficient, timely response to any disaster is the local response. Therefore, Craig said, the most effective long-term recovery of any community is that which is planned and managed at the local level by the impacted community. This is supported in the NDRF (see Box 2), which stresses that federal, state, or other disaster recovery organizations recognize that communities have the lead role in planning for and managing their recovery. Craig noted, however, that in their efforts to "vigorously support local, state, and tribal governments," these agencies and organizations can sometimes provide too much help that may not be consistent with the impacted community's direction.

The NDRF also acknowledges the notion that you cannot, or perhaps should not, always rebuild in exactly the same way as before the disaster. The framework states that successful recovery may involve relocation of some or all of the community's assets (see Box 2).

BOX 2
National Disaster Recovery Framework Excerpts

Leadership and Local Primacy
"Successful recovery requires informed and coordinated leadership throughout all levels of government, sectors of society, and phases of the recovery process. It recognizes that local, State and Tribal governments have ***primary responsibility for the recovery of their communities and play the lead role in planning for and managing all aspects of community recovery. This is a basic, underlying principle that should not be overlooked by State, Federal and other disaster recovery managers.*** States act in support of their communities, evaluate their capabilities, and provide a means of support for overwhelmed local governments. The Federal Government is a partner and facilitator in recovery, prepared to enlarge its role when the disaster impacts relate to areas where Federal jurisdiction is primary or affects national security. The Federal Government, while acknowledging the primary role of local, State and Tribal governments, is prepared to vigorously support local, State and Tribal governments in a large-scale disaster or catastrophic incident." (FEMA, 2011, pp. 9-10 [emphasis added])

Achieving Disaster Recovery

"Recovery is more than the community's return to pre-disaster circumstances, especially when the community determines that these circumstances are no longer sustainable, competitive or functional as shown by the community's post-disaster condition. A successful recovery in this case *may include a decision to relocate all or some portion of the community assets* and restoration of the affected area to a more natural environment. In these circumstances, the community recovery decision making is informed by evaluating all alternatives and options and avoiding simple rebuilding or reconstructing of an area that continues to be vulnerable." (FEMA, 2011, p. 13 [emphasis added])

SOURCE: Craig presentation (February 23, 2012) citing FEMA (2011).

Planning for the Unexpected

As an example of the importance of thorough long-term recovery planning, Craig shared his experiences as the incident manager for the health and medical state responses for Hurricane Katrina in Mississippi. The Gulf Coast Medical Center in Biloxi, Mississippi, was a 189-bed hospital directly across the street from the beach. Destroyed by the hurricane, the hospital reopened with limited services in 2006. Inpatient services dropped by 40 percent, and the hospital closed again on January 1, 2008. Much of the surrounding population had moved north, Craig explained, and few were left to accommodate with health services in that location. In other words, the hospital did not close in 2008 as a direct result of the storm, but closed because planning was probably inadequate at the community level to foresee that the community would relocate and that the hospital, rebuilt in place, would no longer be central to its users. The current plan is for the hospital to relocate north to follow the population shift. Other components of the health care system, such as pharmacies and physician offices, also moved north to where the people now live, and there is no reason to have a hospital where there are no doctors, patients, or pharmacies.

Another item that was misjudged in the planning was the capacity of the mental health component that would be needed. Around 40 percent of Mississippians in the lower part of the three counties on the coast had either signed up for, were currently in, or had recently completed mental health services, but this was not sufficiently planned. Moving forward, plans need to address the ability to maintain capacity of critical mental health services for effected populations.

In addition, following the hurricane the population density shifted so that more individuals are now living inland. Therefore, the active recovery effort is having to focus on developing a new regional water and wastewater infrastructure further inland to provide service to the relocated population. Overall, the relocation of the population to a less-vulnerable area was a critical factor in recovery, but was unplanned.

Craig stressed that everyone, including local businesses, should have long-term recovery planning. As an example, he described a current challenge facing the recovery efforts following the EF-5 tornado in Smithville, Michigan, in 2011. More than 150 homes, nearly all of the businesses, all of the city government, the funeral home, and the Piggly Wiggly were destroyed. The Piggly Wiggly was the only grocery store in Smithville. The parent company is concerned about rebuilding in Smithville because it does not know if the people will come back. In turn, people are hesitant to come back until they find out if the Piggly Wiggly is reopening.

The last example Craig shared related to the historic flood impacting 14 counties in Mississippi in 2011, displacing thousands of residents and destroying thousands of acres of farmland, with an estimated crop loss of around $800 million. During the response phase, the state created a health care flood impact taskforce of interested parties from the health care systems in those 14 counties (e.g., pharmacies, physician groups, the state medical association, the hospital association, long-term care, hospice, home health care). The taskforce composed of local impacted communities continued through the short-term recovery and worked together to assist in planning for the long term. This became a best practice. The next step is to form official regional health care coalitions out of the taskforce, and possibly a multiagency coordinating system. Emergency plans for many hazards in this particular event were insufficient, Craig said, and through this coalition there is now a better opportunity to coordinate and plan locally.

Depth and Breadth of Local Recovery Planning and Priority Setting

A participant commented that from a community perspective, engaging in recovery planning can look very daunting. There are ancillary services that are critical for health care, such as public and private emergency medical service (EMS) units, contracted hospital linen services, water, power, and a host of other suppliers. Such services also cross local or state borders, so planning may involve multiple states, commonwealths, or jurisdictions. How necessary is it, for example, to find out the details of one specific hospital relying on one set of specific suppliers and another hospital relying on other entities?

The HHS Hospital Preparedness Program emphasizes the development of coalitions both in and outside hospitals, including EMS, individual providers, long-term skilled nursing facilities, and other community members, Yeskey responded. He noted that hospitals are likely to be competitors on a day-to-day basis, so bringing them together to work cooperatively and discuss their systems with competitors can be challenging. It is important to share protocols and work out the details in advance regarding resources and staff. For example, if one hospital loans nurses to another, who will pay their salary? If a ventilator is loaned out and ends up getting transferred out of the state due to patient transfer, who is covering the reimbursement? Eventually one needs to work down to this level of detail, Yeskey said, but it does not all have to be done in 1 day.

Priorities in any response situation, Yeskey said, are to save lives, protect the public's health, protect responders, protect infrastructure, and maintain situational awareness. Each community needs to determine its own priorities for recovery, for example, the order of priority for recovery of public utilities, debris removal, law enforcement, health care, or education. Making this determination in advance will help significantly with preparedness, response, and recovery of the community.

Craig added that the people and the partnerships are almost as important as the plan. In his experience, strong leadership in the development of the vision for where the long-term recovery is going and inclusion of all key stakeholders is what leads to success. Without that leadership and without all of the right people, what looks like a perfect solution very quickly falls apart.

BARRIERS AND CHALLENGES TO RECOVERY

A key challenge to response and recovery is creating national policies and making national decisions that translate well to the local levels. For a private-sector partner, a major challenge when dealing with a national public health response is having corporate solutions that can be applied across the country. A national and global retailer such as Target needs national and global strategies, Riff said. In response to the

H1N1 influenza pandemic, for example, 1,744 Target locations had vaccine available for the healthy public. The company has one standing protocol for how to give vaccinations. What Riff found, however, was that in dealing with state and county health departments, there were about 1,500 vaccination protocols and communication campaigns, which made it challenging to execute on the company's national strategy.

Another challenge Riff highlighted is getting communities to partner with the private sector ahead of time to participate in planning, instead of calling for supplies after the disaster. Craig concurred that, at the local and state levels, planning efforts are not engaging the private sector to the extent needed. There is a general hesitancy to leverage and use both the private sector and NGOs. But the government does not have enough resources to handle disasters alone, and may not be the most efficient in response, commented Craig. Private industry can often mobilize much faster than government, sometimes delivering supplies within hours, while a government response may take days.

Situational awareness and "rumor control" are also challenges. Information changes over the course of time, impacting decision making, Yeskey said. When a policy changes due to new information, sometimes it is viewed as indecision. For example, when a case of H1N1 influenza shuts down a school, and it is then learned that the situation is not as severe as initially thought, so the policy changes and the school reopens, it is difficult to convey to the public that we know what we are doing, he said. Based on what is known at the time, the best protective decisions and policies are put forth, and are likely to change based on new information. Communicating this is a significant challenge.

Ingram noted that a challenge for FEMA is getting local communities to pay attention to the NDRF pre-disaster. Communities are already overwhelmed, and there is some denial that they need to prepare. Post-disaster, there is much interest in planning for the next time, but we need to convey the importance of pre-disaster planning, and to find those champions in the communities that can help the process. Working together before a disaster is challenging, MacIntyre agreed, especially as public health positions continue to be cut and finding the time to forge the needed relationships becomes very difficult.

An obstacle to planning, Craig added, is that some states have a certificate-of-need process. Health care planners at the state level must be convinced that resources are needed in different places before capital projects can be approved.

FINAL REMARKS

Each long-term recovery is different and unique, and planning for all of the variables of a recovery is very difficult, Craig noted. At the federal level, FEMA and HHS have key coordination and support roles, bringing money and people to recovery operations. State government helps to ensure that the local government and community get the support they need for their long-term recovery. The local community has the lead role in planning for and managing all aspects of community recovery. State and local governments need to ensure that their plan works for their community and engages the private sector and all of the parts of the health care system.

REFERENCE

FEMA (Federal Emergency Management Administration). 2011. *National Disaster Recovery Framework.* http://www.fema.gov/pdf/recoveryframework/ndrfpdf (accessed April 13, 2012).

A

Workshop Statement of Task

An ad hoc planning committee will plan and conduct a public session in workshop format at the 2012 Preparedness Summit that will examine the long-term recovery of the U.S. health care service delivery infrastructure. This session will feature invited presentations and discussions that will provide participants with an opportunity to engage representatives from federal, state, and local governments as well as the nonprofit and private sectors to identify services necessary to maintain or improve the affected health care service delivery infrastructure necessary to meet the long-term physical and behavioral health needs of affected populations. The discussions will highlight lessons learned from previous disasters, and focus on opportunities to leverage programs and activities across the public, private, and nonprofit sectors that support long-term recovery and mass casualty care. Specifically, presentations and discussions will

- Identify services necessary to maintain or improve the affected health care service delivery infrastructure to ensure it meets the long-term physical and behavioral health needs of affected populations.
- Discuss the roles and functions of the relevant emergency support functions in facilitating long-term recovery of the health care service delivery infrastructure.
- Highlight lessons learned from previous disasters, and identify priorities for pre-incident operational plans, with a specific focus on opportunities to leverage programs and activities across the public, private, and nonprofit sectors that support long-term recovery and mass casualty care.

The committee will develop the agenda for the workshop session, select and invite speakers and discussants, and moderate the discussions. An individually authored workshop summary will be prepared based on the information gathered and the discussions held during the workshop session.

B

Agenda

SESSION DESCRIPTION

Well beyond the initial response to a disaster, the long-term recovery of the health care service delivery infrastructure requires a broad public-private partnership. This long-term recovery is facilitated primarily through FEMA and in conjunction with HHS's ESF #8 responsibilities. This town hall session will allow participants an opportunity to engage representatives from federal, state, and local governments, emergency management and public health, and the nonprofit and private sectors to identify services necessary to maintain or improve the affected health care service delivery infrastructure to ensure it meets the long-term physical and behavioral health needs of affected populations. The town hall session will also engage state and local authorities in a dialog around their needs and will be an opportunity for input about how these needs can potentially be addressed through the relevant ESF policies and guidance documents. The discussions will highlight lessons learned from previous disasters, and identify priorities for pre-incident operational plans, with a specific focus on opportunities to leverage programs and activities across the public, private, and nonprofit sectors that support long-term recovery and mass casualty care.

LEARNING OBJECTIVES

- Identify services necessary to maintain or improve the affected health care service delivery infrastructure to ensure it meets the long-term physical and behavioral health needs of affected populations.

- Discuss the roles and functions of the relevant emergency support functions in facilitating long-term recovery of the health care service delivery infrastructure.
- Highlight lessons learned from previous disasters, and identify priorities for pre-incident operational plans, with a specific focus on opportunities to leverage programs and activities across the public, private, and nonprofit sectors that support long-term recovery and mass casualty care.

Lynne Kidder, *Session Chair*
President
Bipartisan WMD Terrorism Research Center

Panelists:

Deborah Ingram
Assistant Administrator
Recovery Directorate
Office of Response & Recovery
DHS/FEMA

Kevin Yeskey
Deputy Assistant Secretary
HHS/ASPR

Josh Riff
Medical Director
Target

Linda MacIntyre
National Chair, Red Cross Nursing
Assistant Clinical Professor, UCSF

James Craig
Director, Office of Health Protection
Mississippi State Department of Health

C

Speaker Biographies

Lynn Kidder, M.A., B.A. (*Session Chair*), is the president and chief executive officer of the Bipartisan WMD Terrorism Research Center (the WMD Center), a not-for-profit research and educational organization, founded by former senators Bob Graham and Jim Talent at the conclusion of the Congressional Commission on the Prevention of Weapons of Mass Destruction, Proliferation, and Terrorism. The WMD Center was chartered to help government and private-sector leaders better understand the unique threats and challenges of bioterrorism and the actions required for effective response to either deliberate or naturally occurring biological disasters. She was the principal investigator for the WMD Center's 2011 Bio-Response Report Card. Ms. Kidder also serves as a senior advisor to the Center for Excellence in Disaster Management and Humanitarian Assistance, a Department of Defense organization based at U.S. Pacific Command. It provides training to enhance civil-military, interagency, and NGO coordination during international disaster response. Ms. Kidder was formerly a senior vice president at Business Executives for National Security, where she led the development and nationwide implementation of programs to facilitate resilience-focused public-private collaboration. Ms. Kidder's other professional experience includes executive-level management in state government, corporate government affairs, and 8 years as a professional staff member in the U.S. Senate. She also served for 5 years as the executive director for the nonprofit North Bay Leadership Council in Northern California, and was credited with numerous regional initiatives among private employers, public officials, and other civic leaders. She holds a B.A. from Indiana University and a master's degree from the University of Texas at Austin, and did postgraduate study in public administration at George Mason University.

James Craig was named health protection director at the Mississippi State Department of Health in 2004 after serving as its director of the Office of Emergency Planning and Response for the agency. Prior to this position, he served as the director of Emergency Medical Services. He was recruited to the agency in 1992 from Louisiana Health and Hospitals, Emergency Medical Services Division. Protecting the public has been a significant part of his life. He served as chair of the Mississippi Fire Fighters Minimum Standards and Training Board. He is also an emergency medical technician, hazardous material technician, and volunteer fire chief in his local community. Mr. Craig has an A.A.S. in forensic science from Louisiana State University and a B.S. in industrial technology/occupational safety from the University of Southwestern Louisiana.

Deborah Ingram, M.A., is the assistant administrator, Recovery Directorate at FEMA. Her public service career spans more than 30 years and includes broad experience in a variety of programs at the federal and local government levels. For more than 10 years, Ms. Ingram has served in a number of senior positions in FEMA's headquarters. In her capacity as assistant administrator, Ms. Ingram has responsibility for leadership and oversight of mandated federal disaster assistance programs that support individuals and communities affected by disasters in their efforts to recover, including individual assistance, public assistance, community recovery, and mass care and voluntary agency coordination. These programs constitute the majority of the resources provided by the federal government (through FEMA) to directly address the short-, medium-, and long-term impacts of a disaster on individuals and communities. Previously, Ms. Ingram held a variety of senior positions in FEMA's Federal Insurance and Mitigation Directorate, where she was responsible for programs that assist states, tribes, and local communities to reduce their risk to natural hazards and disasters. Among her many achievements, Ms. Ingram was instrumental in leading the unification of hazard mitigation grant programs, building strong relationships with FEMA's partners, and, during the summer of 2010, providing key leadership in development and support of the Integrated Services Team during the aftermath of the Deepwater Horizon oil spill. Ms. Ingram was appointed to the federal Senior Executive Service in 2007. Prior to coming to FEMA,

Ms. Ingram spent 11 years at the Environmental Protection Agency, where she held a variety of senior and management positions in strategic planning and administration and resources management. Ms. Ingram started her public service career working at the local government level in North Carolina, and later in Virginia, where she managed and implemented a variety of federally funded grant programs. Ms. Ingram holds a B.S. in psychology from East Carolina University, an M.A. in public administration from the University of Virginia, and an M.A. in psychology from George Mason University.

Linda MacIntyre, B.S.N., Ph.D., is chair of the American Red Cross National Nursing Committee, and an assistant professor at the University of California, San Francisco. After working as a residential social worker in England, Dr. MacIntyre worked briefly on a medical surgical/oncology floor before moving to Missouri, where she was a hemodialysis nurse for 5 years. Working in hemodialysis was the impetus for Dr. MacIntyre to move into a position to address health prevention, and this led her to become the community health nurse manager and later the director of community health and youth for the Greater Kansas City Chapter of the American Red Cross. She was responsible for health screening programs, HIV and AIDS education, Family Caregiving Training, youth programs, a large flu shot program, and local disaster health preparedness and response. Under her direction, the flu shot program grew from serving 4,000 to as many as 18,500 in 1 year. Dr. MacIntyre worked closely with community agencies and the Kansas City public health department in addressing rates of HIV and AIDS. She coordinated culturally specific HIV and AIDS training for African American and Hispanic communities in partnership with multiple agencies, the incidence of HIV and AIDS decreased in African American and Hispanic individuals in the Greater Kansas City Area.

Dr. MacIntyre participated in community coalitions and worked on an NIH Community Disaster Information System project based at Miami University in Ohio. She served on several community coalitions, was a member of the Medical Reserve Corps Steering Committee for an eight-county region, and worked closely with the public health department to improve disaster response in the greater Kansas City metropolitan area. Dr. MacIntyre was a member of the Red Cross National Nursing Committee and worked extensively on a committee that addressed pharmaceutical stockpiling and delivery strategies related to disaster preparedness and response. As a volunteer, she worked as the American Red Cross Pacific

Service Area Health Care Professional Liaison to develop partnerships between schools of nursing and local chapters in promoting health education and disaster preparedness. Dr. MacIntyre attended state Public Health Advisory Committee meetings, helped develop strategic plans, and provided consultation on influenza pandemic preparation. Dr. MacIntyre earned a first-class honors degree in theology form Westminster College in Oxford, England, her nursing degree from Texas Christian University, and her Ph.D. in nursing from the University of California, San Francisco.

Joshua Riff, M.D., M.B.A., is the medical director of Target Corporation and is a board-certified emergency medicine physician. After medical school he completed his residency in emergency medicine at Johns Hopkins Hospital, where he learned of the plight of an inner-city health care system and the value of alternative models of health care delivery. Upon graduation he moved to Tucson Medical Center, where he worked in an emergency room, seeing over 100,000 patients per year. His experience there taught him the difficulties associated with access to high-quality medical care and of the need for an integrated medical system. In 2006 he started at Target as medical director of Target Clinics, where he helped to provide access to convenient, affordable, and high-quality medical care through health clinics located in Target stores. Currently, he is medical director of Target Corporation where he plays a role in helping to create a culture of health and wellness for Target's more than 350,000 employees; reinforcing the retailer as a leading partner in health care to consumers; and ensuring the company's preparedness for influenza pandemics or other public health needs. Dr. Riff sits on the editorial board for the Center for Infectious Disease Research and Policy and *Retail Clinic News*. He is a member of the Hennepin County Medical Foundation and sits on the National Business Group on Health Evidence Based Benefit Design committee. He completed his M.D./M.B.A. at Tufts University in conjunction with Brandeis University in Boston, Massachusetts. During this time he started the M.D./M.B.A. consulting group in which students work on hospital consulting projects ranging from ideal staffing levels to waiting time analyses.

Kevin Yeskey, M.D., is acting director of the Office of Preparedness and Emergency Operations and acting deputy assistant secretary in the Office of Public Health Emergency Preparedness, HHS. He is an associate professor and former director of the Center for Disaster and Humanitarian

Assistance Medicine at the Uniformed Services University of the Health Sciences (USUHS) School of Medicine. He held a variety of disaster response positions while on active duty with the U.S. Public Health Service before retiring in 2003. Dr. Yeskey also served as senior medical policy advisor in FEMA's Emergency Management Agency's Response Division and was director of the Office of Emergency Response for HHS. From 1999 to 2002, he was assigned to the Centers for Disease Control and Prevention and served as director of the Bioterrorism Preparedness and Response Program at the National Center for Infectious Diseases. Before that, he was associate director for Emergency Public Health and Science in the Division of Emergency and Environmental Health Services at the National Center for Environmental Health. For 16 years, he was a medical officer on the U.S. Public Health Service Disaster Medical Assistance Team, 6 years as commanding officer. Dr. Yeskey also served as chief of medical operations for the Kosovo refugee crisis at Fort Dix, New Jersey. He was a member of a four-person federal health assessment team that assisted with the response to the Oklahoma City bombing. Dr. Yeskey received his undergraduate degree from Brown University and his medical degree from USUHS, and is board certified in emergency medicine.